Thriving Through Change

Your Essential Guide to Navigating Menopause with Wellness

Aria Vitality

DEDICATION

To all those who strive for inner peace, balance, and well-being amidst life's myriad challenges. Your courage, resilience, and commitment to personal growth inspire the pages of this book. May these words serve as a guiding light on your journey towards a harmonious and fulfilled life.

CONTENTS

ACKNOWLEDGMENTS

This book is the culmination of collective wisdom, support, and encouragement from numerous individuals and resources. I extend my deepest gratitude to all those who have contributed to its creation.

To my family and friends, thank you for your unwavering love, patience, and understanding throughout this endeavor. Your support has been my anchor during moments of doubt and inspiration during times of creativity.

I am indebted to the mental health professionals whose expertise and dedication have shaped the content of this book. Your commitment to helping others navigate the complexities of the mind is truly commendable.

To the readers who embark on this journey of self-discovery and growth, thank you for entrusting me with your time and attention. It is my sincere hope that the insights shared within these pages resonate with you and empower you to cultivate a life of balance, resilience, and fulfillment.

Finally, I extend my heartfelt appreciation to the team at SmartWave Research Group, whose professionalism, guidance, and enthusiasm have brought this project to fruition.

With deep appreciation,
Aria Vitality

CHAPTER 1

UNDERSTANDING MENOPAUSE

Menopause – a word that can evoke a range of emotions in women, from confusion and anxiety to relief and liberation. But what exactly is menopause, and why is it such a significant transition in a woman's life?

1.1 What is Menopause?

Menopause is the natural end of a woman's reproductive years. It's marked by the permanent cessation of menstruation for at least 12 consecutive months, not due to pregnancy or other health conditions. This occurs when the ovaries significantly decrease their production of estrogen and progesterone, hormones that play a crucial role in regulating the menstrual cycle and other bodily functions.

Think of menopause as a graduation ceremony – you're officially done with the chapter of childbearing, but a whole new chapter filled with potential and self-discovery awaits.

1.2 The Stages of Menopause: Perimenopause, Menopause, and Postmenopause

Menopause isn't a single event; it's a process that unfolds in several stages:

- **Perimenopause:** This is the lead-up to menopause, typically lasting several years (although it can vary from woman to woman). During perimenopause, your ovaries gradually start producing less estrogen and progesterone, leading to fluctuations in hormone levels. This can cause a variety of symptoms, including irregular periods, hot flashes, mood swings, and sleep disturbances.

- **Menopause:** This is the official marker of the end of your menstrual cycle. Menopause is confirmed when you haven't had a period for 12 consecutive months, not due to other factors.

- **Postmenopause:** This stage begins after menopause and continues for the rest of your life. During this time, your body adjusts to the low hormone levels and the symptoms you may have experienced during perimenopause may improve or lessen. However, some women may still experience certain symptoms like vaginal dryness or changes in sleep patterns.

Understanding these stages can help you navigate the transition and recognize the various changes your body might be experiencing.

1.3 Common Symptoms of Menopause

The hormonal fluctuations during menopause can cause a wide range of symptoms, and the severity and experience will vary for each woman. Some of the most common symptoms include:

- **Hot flashes and night sweats:** These are sudden feelings of intense heat that can cause flushing of the skin, sweating, and a racing heart. They are a hallmark symptom of menopause and can be quite disruptive to sleep and daily activities.
- **Irregular periods:** As your estrogen levels decline, your periods may become irregular, lighter, or heavier than usual. Eventually, they will stop

altogether.

- **Vaginal dryness:** Due to decreased estrogen levels, the vaginal tissues can become thinner and less lubricated, leading to discomfort during intercourse and increased risk of urinary tract infections.

- **Sleep disturbances:** Difficulty falling asleep, waking frequently during the night, and waking up feeling unrested are common complaints during menopause.

- **Mood swings:** Fluctuations in estrogen can affect brain chemicals that regulate mood, leading to irritability, anxiety, and even depression.

- **Changes in memory and concentration:** Some women may experience difficulty concentrating, forgetfulness, or "brain fog" during menopause. This is usually temporary and may improve with lifestyle modifications.

- **Reduced libido:** Lower estrogen levels can affect sexual desire and arousal.

- **Changes in physical appearance:** You may notice changes in your body shape, such as weight gain around the abdomen, and thinning hair.

It's important to remember that not every woman will experience all of these symptoms, and the severity can vary greatly. However, if any symptoms are significantly impacting your quality of life, it's important to talk to your doctor. They can help you manage your symptoms and ensure you're on the right track for overall well-being during this transition.

CHAPTER 2

THE HORMONAL SHIFT

Menopause is a symphony of change orchestrated by a shift in the hormonal landscape. Understanding the key players and how their levels fluctuate during this transition is crucial to navigating the physical and emotional changes you might experience.

2.1 Estrogen and Progesterone: The Key Players

Two main hormones take center stage during your reproductive years: estrogen and progesterone. They work together in a beautiful dance to regulate your menstrual cycle, prepare your body for pregnancy, and influence various bodily functions.

- **Estrogen:** This multifaceted hormone plays a vital role in regulating your menstrual cycle, promoting healthy bone density, maintaining vaginal tissue health, and even influencing mood and cognitive function.

- **Progesterone:** This hormone works hand-in-hand with estrogen, preparing the uterine lining for pregnancy and regulating the menstrual cycle.

Throughout your reproductive years, estrogen and progesterone levels rise and fall in a predictable pattern, dictating the different phases of your menstrual cycle.

2.2 How Hormonal Changes Affect Your Body

As you approach perimenopause, your ovaries gradually start producing less estrogen and progesterone. This decline disrupts the delicate hormonal balance, leading to a domino effect on various bodily functions. Here's how these changes might manifest:

- **Menstrual Cycle Irregularities:** Fluctuating hormone levels during perimenopause can cause your periods to become irregular, lighter, or heavier than usual. Eventually, as estrogen levels drop significantly, ovulation ceases, and menstruation stops altogether.
- **Hot Flashes and Night Sweats:** A decrease in

estrogen disrupts the body's temperature regulation system, leading to the sudden feeling of intense heat, flushing of the skin, and sweating associated with hot flashes. These can be quite disruptive to sleep, causing night sweats and leaving you feeling exhausted.

- **Vaginal Dryness and Changes in Sexual Function:** Estrogen plays a crucial role in maintaining the health and lubrication of vaginal tissues. As estrogen levels decline, these tissues become thinner and less lubricated, leading to vaginal dryness and discomfort during intercourse. Reduced libido and decreased sexual arousal can also occur due to hormonal changes.

- **Bone Density and Increased Risk of Osteoporosis:** Estrogen plays a vital role in maintaining bone density. The decrease in estrogen after menopause puts women at a higher risk of developing osteoporosis, a condition that weakens bones and increases the risk of fractures.

- **Mood Swings and Changes in Brain Function:** Estrogen receptors are present in areas of the brain that regulate mood and cognitive function.

Fluctuations in estrogen levels can affect these brain chemicals, leading to symptoms like irritability, anxiety, mood swings, and even difficulty concentrating or remembering things (often referred to as "brain fog").

It's important to note that the severity and experience of these changes will vary greatly from woman to woman. Some women may sail through menopause with minimal symptoms, while others may experience a more pronounced impact.

2.3 The Long-Term Health Impact of Menopause

While menopause can bring a variety of changes in the short term, it's also important to consider the long-term health implications. Here are some key points to remember:

- **Increased Risk of Heart Disease:** Estrogen has a protective effect on the cardiovascular system. After menopause, the risk of heart disease increases for women.
- **Changes in Body Fat Distribution:** You may notice

a shift in how your body stores fat. With declining estrogen levels, fat tends to accumulate more around the abdomen (visceral fat) compared to the hips and thighs (subcutaneous fat) which was more common during your reproductive years. Visceral fat is linked to an increased risk of heart disease and other chronic conditions.

- **Importance of Bone Health:** As mentioned earlier, the decline in estrogen puts women at a higher risk of osteoporosis. Taking steps to maintain strong bones through diet, exercise, and potentially consulting your doctor about bone density scans and medication options is crucial for long-term health.

Understanding these long-term health considerations can empower you to prioritize healthy lifestyle choices and potentially discuss preventative measures with your doctor during your menopause transition.

Remember, menopause is not a disease; it's a natural biological transition. By understanding the hormonal shifts and their impact on your body, you can take proactive steps to manage your symptoms, maintain your overall well-being, and thrive during this exciting new chapter of your life.

CHAPTER 3

TAMING THE TIDE: MANAGING HOT FLASHES AND NIGHT
SWEATS

Hot flashes and night sweats – these are some of the most common and disruptive symptoms associated with menopause. They can be incredibly frustrating, interrupting sleep, affecting your daily activities, and leaving you feeling flushed and uncomfortable. But fear not! There are ways to manage these fiery waves and reclaim your cool.

3.1 What are Hot Flashes and Night Sweats?

Hot flashes are a sudden feeling of intense heat that washes over your upper body and face. This sensation can be accompanied by flushing of the skin, sweating, a racing heart, and even chills once the wave passes. Night sweats are essentially hot flashes that occur during sleep, often leaving you drenched in sweat and disrupting your sleep quality.

These symptoms occur because of the decline in estrogen

levels during menopause. Estrogen helps regulate your body's internal temperature. When estrogen levels drop, your body's ability to regulate temperature becomes less precise, leading to the sudden surges of heat associated with hot flashes.

3.2 Lifestyle Modifications for Reducing Hot Flashes

The good news is that several lifestyle modifications can help you manage the frequency and intensity of hot flashes:

- **Dress in layers:** This allows you to easily adjust to temperature changes. Opt for breathable, natural fabrics like cotton or linen.
- **Stay cool:** Avoid triggers that can induce hot flashes, such as spicy foods, hot beverages, caffeine, and alcohol. Keep your environment cool by using fans or air conditioning at night.
- **Manage stress:** Stress can worsen hot flashes. Relaxation techniques such as deep breathing exercises, meditation, or yoga can be helpful.
- **Maintain a healthy weight:** Excess weight can contribute to hot flashes. A balanced diet and regular

exercise can help manage your weight and potentially reduce hot flash frequency.

- **Sleep hygiene:** Establishing a regular sleep schedule and practicing good sleep hygiene can help improve sleep quality, even if you experience night sweats.

3.3 Exploring Complementary Therapies for Relief

While lifestyle modifications can be very effective, some women may seek additional support for managing hot flashes. Here are some complementary therapies worth exploring:

- **Acupuncture:** This traditional Chinese medicine practice involves inserting thin needles into specific points on the body. Studies suggest acupuncture may offer some relief from hot flashes.

- **Hypnosis:** Hypnotherapy can help you manage your body's response to triggers that initiate hot flashes.

- **Herbal remedies:** Certain herbs, such as black cohosh or red clover, are sometimes used to manage menopausal symptoms, though research on their effectiveness is ongoing. It's important to consult with your doctor before using any herbal remedies to ensure they are safe and don't interact with any medications you're taking.

- **Cognitive-behavioral therapy (CBT):** CBT can help you develop coping mechanisms to manage stress and anxiety, which can exacerbate hot flashes.

Remember, every woman's experience with hot flashes is unique. Experiment with different strategies to find what works best for you. Don't hesitate to discuss your concerns and preferences with your doctor. They can help you create a personalized plan to manage your hot flashes and night sweats effectively.

CHAPTER 4

Sleepless Nights No More: Strategies for Better Sleep During Menopause

Ah, sleep – that elusive state we all crave, especially during menopause. Night sweats, hot flashes, and hormonal fluctuations can wreak havoc on your sleep quality, leaving you feeling exhausted and drained. But don't despair! By understanding the connections between menopause and sleep disruption, and by incorporating some key sleep hygiene strategies, you can reclaim those restful nights.

4.1 The Connection Between Menopause and Sleep Disruption

Several factors related to menopause can disrupt your sleep:

- **Hot flashes and night sweats:** These sudden surges of heat and sweating can wake you up abruptly and make it difficult to fall back asleep.

- **Mood swings and anxiety:** Fluctuations in estrogen levels can lead to increased anxiety, making it harder to quiet your mind and drift off to sleep.

- **Changes in body temperature:** Declining estrogen levels can affect your body's natural temperature regulation, making it harder to maintain a cool, comfortable sleep environment.

- **Increased need to urinate:** More frequent urination, especially at night, can disrupt your sleep cycle. This may be due to changes in bladder function or increased fluid intake to cope with night sweats.

4.2 Creating a Sleep-Friendly Environment

The good news is that you can create a sleep sanctuary that promotes better sleep:

- **Temperature control:** Keep your bedroom cool, ideally between 60-67°F (15.5-19.4°C). Utilize fans or air conditioning to maintain a comfortable temperature.

- **Light and darkness:** Ensure your bedroom is dark

and free of light pollution. Invest in blackout curtains or an eye mask to block out any light that might disrupt your sleep.

- **Comfort is key:** Invest in a comfortable mattress and pillows that support your body. Create a relaxing atmosphere with calming scents like lavender or chamomile.

- **Limit electronics:** Avoid using electronic devices like TVs, laptops, and phones in bed. The blue light emitted by these devices can interfere with sleep patterns.

- **Develop a relaxing bedtime routine:** Establish a regular sleep schedule, going to bed and waking up at the same time each day, even on weekends. Wind down before bed with calming activities like reading a book, taking a warm bath, or listening to relaxing music.

4.3 Relaxation Techniques to Promote Sleep

In addition to creating a sleep-friendly environment, relaxation techniques can help quiet your mind and prepare your body for sleep:

- **Deep breathing exercises:** Techniques like diaphragmatic breathing can slow your heart rate, reduce stress, and promote relaxation.

- **Progressive muscle relaxation:** Tense and release different muscle groups throughout your body to release tension and promote calmness.

- **Meditation:** Mindfulness meditation techniques can help focus your attention on the present moment and quiet racing thoughts.

- **Yoga and gentle stretching:** Light yoga or stretching routines before bed can help ease muscle tension and promote relaxation.

Consistency is key. By implementing these strategies and establishing a regular sleep routine, you can gradually improve your sleep quality and wake up feeling refreshed and ready to take on the day.

CHAPTER 5

Menopause isn't just a physical transition; it can also have a significant impact on your emotional well-being. You might experience a rollercoaster of emotions, from feeling irritable and anxious to tearful and overwhelmed. This chapter will explore the reasons behind these mood swings and provide strategies to navigate them effectively.

5.1 Understanding the Emotional Impact of Menopause

Several factors contribute to the emotional changes you may experience during menopause:

- **Hormonal fluctuations:** Declining estrogen and progesterone levels can affect brain chemicals like serotonin and dopamine, which regulate mood. These fluctuations can lead to irritability, anxiety, mood swings, and even depression.

- **Stress:** Menopause can be a stressful time, with

changes in your body, relationships, and work-life balance. This stress can further exacerbate emotional changes.

- **Sleep disturbances:** As discussed in Chapter 4, sleep disruption is common during menopause. Lack of quality sleep can exacerbate symptoms like anxiety and irritability.

- **Life changes:** Menopause often coincides with other life changes such as empty nest syndrome, aging parents, or career transitions. These changes can add to the emotional rollercoaster some women experience during menopause.

It's important to understand that these emotional changes are normal and temporary for most women. However, if you're struggling to cope, there are ways to manage them and prioritize your mental well-being.

5.2 Strategies for Managing Mood Swings

Here are some strategies to help you navigate the emotional ups and downs of menopause:

- **Acknowledge your feelings:** Don't bottle up your

emotions. Talk to a trusted friend, family member, therapist, or doctor about how you're feeling.

- **Maintain a healthy lifestyle:** Eating a balanced diet, exercising regularly, and getting enough sleep can all positively impact your mood. Prioritize activities you enjoy and that promote relaxation.

- **Stress management:** Techniques like deep breathing, meditation, and yoga can help reduce stress and improve emotional regulation.

- **Stay connected with loved ones:** Social connection is crucial for emotional well-being. Spend time with supportive friends and family who make you feel good.

- **Consider therapy:** A therapist can provide valuable support and guidance in managing mood swings and coping with emotional challenges during menopause.

5.3 Prioritizing Mental Health During Menopause

Here are some additional tips for prioritizing your mental health during menopause:

- **Be kind to yourself:** Remember, menopause is a natural transition, not a personal failing. Treat yourself with compassion and understanding.

- **Set realistic expectations:** Don't expect to feel like your younger self every day. Accept that your experiences may be different, and focus on creating a fulfilling and healthy life during this new chapter.

- **Empower yourself with knowledge:** The more you understand about the emotional changes associated with menopause, the better equipped you are to manage them.

- **Don't hesitate to seek professional help:** If your mood swings are severe or interfering with your daily life, don't hesitate to seek professional help from a therapist or doctor. They can offer support, guidance, and potential treatment options if needed.

By prioritizing your mental and emotional well-being during menopause, you can navigate this transition with greater ease and embrace the positive changes it brings

CHAPTER 6

Menopause isn't just about hot flashes and mood swings; it also marks a significant shift in bone health for women. Understanding the changes that occur and implementing strategies to maintain strong bones is crucial for your long-term health and well-being. This chapter will explore the importance of bone health during menopause and equip you with tools to build and maintain a strong foundation for your body.

6.1 Why Bone Health is Crucial During Menopause

Estrogen plays a vital role in maintaining bone density throughout your life. As estrogen levels decline during menopause, this delicate balance is disrupted, leading to a gradual decrease in bone mineral density. This puts women at an increased risk of developing osteoporosis, a condition characterized by weak and brittle bones that are more susceptible to fractures.

Here's why bone health is especially critical during menopause:

- **Increased Risk of Fractures:** Weakened bones due to osteoporosis are more prone to fractures, particularly in the hips, spine, and wrists. These fractures can be debilitating and significantly impact your quality of life.

- **Long-Term Complications:** Fractures can lead to pain, disability, and even loss of independence. In some cases, surgery may be required to repair fractures, adding another layer of stress and recovery time.

The good news is that you can take proactive steps to maintain strong bones and reduce your risk of osteoporosis during menopause and beyond.

6.2 Dietary Strategies for Strong Bones

A healthy diet rich in essential nutrients plays a crucial role in promoting bone health:

- **Calcium:** Calcium is the building block of strong

bones. Aim for adequate daily intake of calcium-rich foods like dairy products, leafy green vegetables, tofu, and fortified foods.

- **Vitamin D:** Vitamin D helps your body absorb calcium from your diet. Include good sources of vitamin D in your diet, such as fatty fish, egg yolks, or consider taking a vitamin D supplement after consulting your doctor.

- **Protein:** Protein is also essential for bone health. Include lean protein sources like fish, chicken, beans, and lentils in your diet.

- **Fruits and vegetables:** A diet rich in fruits and vegetables provides essential vitamins, minerals, and antioxidants that contribute to overall bone health.

- **Limit sodium and processed foods:** Excessive sodium intake can contribute to bone loss. Aim to limit processed foods and added salt in your diet.

Remember, a balanced and nutritious diet is essential for overall health, but consulting a registered dietitian can help you create a personalized plan that addresses your specific needs for bone health during menopause.

6.3 Exercise for Bone Density and Overall Health

Weight-bearing exercises are crucial for building and maintaining strong bones. Here's why exercise is essential:

- **Stimulates bone growth:** Weight-bearing exercises like walking, jogging, dancing, and strength training put stress on your bones, which stimulates them to become denser and stronger.

- **Improves balance and coordination:** Regular exercise can improve your balance and coordination, reducing your risk of falls and fractures.

- **Overall health benefits:** Exercise benefits your overall health by promoting cardiovascular health, muscle strength, and weight management, all of which contribute to maintaining a healthy skeletal system.

Aim for at least 30 minutes of moderate-intensity weight-bearing exercise most days of the week. Combining weight-bearing exercises with balance and flexibility exercises can further optimize your bone health and overall well-being.

Remember, consistency is key! Building and maintaining

bone health is a lifelong process. By incorporating these dietary and exercise strategies into your routine, you can take control of your bone health during menopause and beyond.

CHAPTER 7

BODY CHANGES AND WEIGHT MANAGEMENT

Menopause brings a wave of changes, and your body composition might be one of them. Understanding how menopause affects your metabolism and weight management strategies can empower you to navigate this transition with confidence.

7.1 How Menopause Affects Your Metabolism

As you enter menopause, your metabolism, the rate at which your body burns calories, may start to slow down. This can be attributed to several factors:

- **Decreasing Estrogen Levels:** Estrogen plays a role in regulating metabolism. Declining estrogen levels can lead to a slight decrease in the number of calories your body burns at rest.

- **Changes in Body Composition:** Muscle mass tends to decrease naturally with age, and muscle burns more calories than fat. This shift in body composition can contribute to a slower metabolism.

- **Lifestyle Factors:** Diet, exercise habits, and overall activity levels all play a significant role in your metabolism. Maintaining healthy lifestyle choices during menopause is crucial for weight management.

While a slower metabolism can make weight management more challenging, it's not an insurmountable obstacle. By being mindful of these changes and implementing some key strategies, you can maintain a healthy weight and feel confident in your body throughout menopause.

7.2 Building a Healthy Eating Plan for Menopause

Here's how to create a healthy eating plan that supports your weight management goals during menopause:

- **Focus on Nutrient-Dense Foods:** Prioritize whole grains, fruits, vegetables, and lean protein sources. These foods provide essential nutrients your body needs while keeping you feeling full and satisfied.

- **Portion Control:** Be mindful of portion sizes. Use smaller plates, and focus on slow, mindful eating to avoid overeating.

- **Limit Added Sugars and Refined Carbs:** Excessive intake of sugary drinks, processed foods, and refined carbohydrates can contribute to weight gain and blood sugar fluctuations. Opt for complex carbohydrates like whole grains and limit sugary treats.

- **Healthy Fats are Your Friend:** Don't be afraid of healthy fats! Include healthy fats from sources like avocados, nuts, seeds, and olive oil in your diet. These fats promote satiety and support overall health.

- **Stay Hydrated:** Drinking plenty of water throughout the day can help curb cravings, improve digestion, and support overall well-being.

Remember, a balanced and sustainable approach is key. Consulting a registered dietitian can help you create a personalized eating plan that addresses your specific needs and preferences during menopause.

7.3 Exercise for Weight Management and Muscle Tone

Exercise plays a crucial role in weight management and overall health during menopause:

- **Boosts Metabolism:** Regular physical activity can help increase your metabolism and burn more calories throughout the day.

- **Builds Muscle Mass:** Strength training exercises help you build and maintain muscle mass, which plays a vital role in boosting metabolism and burning calories even at rest.

- **Improves Body Composition:** A combination of cardio and strength training can help you maintain a healthy body composition, minimizing fat gain and promoting muscle tone.

- **Stress Management:** Exercise is a great way to manage stress, which can contribute to weight gain. Physical activity promotes the release of mood-boosting endorphins, leaving you feeling energized and positive.

Aim for at least 150 minutes of moderate-intensity exercise per week, incorporating both cardio and strength training. Find activities you enjoy, whether it's brisk walking, swimming, dancing, or joining a fitness class.

Remember, consistency is key! By adopting a healthy eating plan and incorporating regular exercise into your routine, you can effectively manage your weight during menopause and feel confident and empowered in your own skin.

CHAPTER 8

REIGNITING YOUR INTIMACY

Menopause can bring about changes not just to your body but also to your intimate life. Understanding how these changes can affect your sexuality and exploring strategies to maintain a fulfilling connection with your partner is crucial for a happy and healthy relationship.

8.1 Understanding How Menopause Affects Sexuality

Declining estrogen levels during menopause can impact your sexual experience in several ways:

- **Vaginal Dryness:** A decrease in estrogen can lead to vaginal dryness and thinning of the vaginal tissues. This can cause discomfort during intercourse and decrease libido.

- **Reduced Sexual Arousal:** Estrogen also plays a role in sexual arousal. Lower estrogen levels may make it take longer to become aroused or experience a decrease in natural lubrication.

- **Changes in Body Image:** Menopause can lead to body image changes, and some women may feel less confident about their bodies, impacting their desire for intimacy.

It's important to remember that these changes don't have to define your sex life. With open communication, exploration, and potentially addressing physical changes, you and your partner can maintain a fulfilling and enjoyable intimate connection.

8.2 Communication and Openness for a Fulfilling Sex Life

Communication is key to a healthy sex life during menopause and beyond. Here's how to keep the conversation flowing:

- **Talk to Your Partner:** Openly discuss any changes you're experiencing and how they're affecting your sexuality. Express your needs and desires honestly, and listen attentively to your partner's perspective.
- **Explore Together:** Be open to exploring new ways

of achieving intimacy. Focus on foreplay, communication, and creating a sensual atmosphere. Don't be afraid to experiment and discover what works best for you as a couple during this new phase.

- **Maintain Physical Intimacy:** Physical touch is essential for intimacy. Cuddling, holding hands, and non-sexual touching can maintain closeness and strengthen your emotional connection.

Remember, menopause doesn't have to mark the end of a fulfilling sex life. By communicating openly and exploring new possibilities together, you and your partner can create a deeply satisfying and intimate connection throughout your lives.

8.3 Exploring Solutions for Vaginal Dryness

Vaginal dryness is a common complaint during menopause. Here are some solutions to explore:

- **Lubricants:** Over-the-counter lubricants can help alleviate vaginal dryness and discomfort during intercourse. Opt for water-based lubricants that are safe for use with condoms.

- **Moisturizers:** Vaginal moisturizers can help maintain moisture and improve the health of vaginal tissues. Consult your doctor before using any vaginal moisturizers.

- **Hormone Replacement Therapy (HRT):** If other solutions aren't sufficient, HRT may be an option for some women. HRT can help replenish estrogen levels and potentially alleviate symptoms like vaginal dryness. However, HRT comes with potential risks and side effects, so discuss it thoroughly with your doctor to determine if it's the right choice for you.

Remember, addressing vaginal dryness can significantly improve your sexual experience during menopause. Don't hesitate to talk to your doctor about solutions that can help you maintain a healthy and enjoyable sex life.

By embracing open communication, exploring new possibilities, and addressing potential physical changes, you can navigate the intimate aspects of menopause with confidence and maintain a fulfilling and passionate connection with your partner.

CHAPTER 9

Championing Your Wellbeing: Self-Care During Menopause

Menopause is a significant transition, and prioritizing self-care is essential for navigating this journey with grace and empowerment. This chapter will explore the importance of self-care, equip you with relaxation techniques for stress management, and highlight the value of building a strong support system for emotional well-being.

9.1 The Importance of Self-Care During Transition

During menopause, your body and mind are undergoing significant changes. Prioritizing self-care allows you to nurture your physical and emotional needs, promoting overall well-being and resilience during this transition.

Here's how self-care benefits you during menopause:

- **Reduces Stress:** Taking time for yourself helps

manage stress, which can exacerbate symptoms like hot flashes and mood swings.

- **Improves Sleep Quality:** Relaxation techniques and a focus on self-care can contribute to better sleep quality, leaving you feeling more energized and resilient.

- **Boosts Mood and Well-Being:** Prioritizing activities you enjoy can elevate your mood, promote feelings of relaxation, and enhance your overall sense of well-being.

- **Empowers You to Take Charge:** Self-care allows you to prioritize your needs and take control of your health during this transition.

By incorporating self-care practices into your routine, you can navigate menopause with greater ease and embrace the positive changes it brings.

9.2 Relaxation Techniques for Stress Management

Stress can significantly impact your experience of menopause. Here are some relaxation techniques to incorporate into your self-care routine:

- **Deep Breathing Exercises:** Techniques like diaphragmatic breathing can slow your heart rate, promote relaxation, and reduce stress. Focus on slow, deep breaths from your abdomen, feeling your belly rise and fall with each inhalation and exhalation.

- **Meditation:** Mindfulness meditation techniques can help you focus on the present moment and quiet racing thoughts. There are many guided meditations available online or through apps to help you get started.

- **Progressive Muscle Relaxation:** Tense and release different muscle groups throughout your body to release tension and promote relaxation. Start by tensing your toes, hold for a few seconds, then release and feel the relaxation spread through your body. Repeat with different muscle groups, working your way up your body.

- **Yoga and Gentle Stretching:** Light yoga or stretching routines can help ease muscle tension and promote relaxation. Focus on gentle movements and deep breaths as you move through your stretches.

Find relaxation techniques that resonate with you and incorporate them into your daily routine. Even a few minutes of focused relaxation can make a significant difference in managing stress and promoting overall well-being during menopause.

9.3 Building a Support System for Emotional Well-being

A strong support system is crucial for navigating the emotional ups and downs of menopause. Surround yourself with positive and supportive people who validate your feelings and encourage you throughout this transition.

Here's how to build a supportive network:

- **Connect with Friends and Family:** Spend time with loved ones who make you feel good about yourself. Talk openly about your experiences and lean on them for support.

- **Consider a Menopause Support Group:** Connecting with other women experiencing similar changes can be incredibly valuable. Support groups offer a safe space to share experiences, learn from one another, and feel less alone.

- **Talk to Your Doctor:** Your doctor is a valuable resource for information and support. Don't hesitate to discuss your concerns and explore treatment options if necessary.

- **Consider Therapy:** A therapist can provide a safe space to discuss your emotional challenges and develop coping mechanisms for managing stress and mood swings.

Building a strong support system allows you to feel heard, understood, and empowered during menopause. Don't hesitate to reach out and connect with the people who can support you on this journey.

Menopause is a natural transition, not a disease. By prioritizing self-care, incorporating relaxation techniques, and building a strong support system, you can navigate this chapter with grace, maintain your well-being, and thrive in the years to come.

CHAPTER 10

EMBRACING THE NEW YOU: MENOPAUSE AND BEYOND

Menopause marks the end of your reproductive years, but it certainly doesn't signal the end of your vitality, health, or happiness. This chapter aims to empower you to reframe menopause as a positive transition and equip you with the knowledge and resources to live a vibrant and fulfilling life in the years to come.

10.1 Reframing Menopause as a Positive Change

Menopause can be viewed as a liberation from the physical demands of the menstrual cycle. It's a time to focus on your overall well-being and celebrate the wisdom and experience you've accumulated. Here's a shift in perspective:

- **Freedom from Periods:** No more cramps, bloating, or PMS! Embrace the newfound hormonal stability and predictability.

- **Focus on Self-Care:** Prioritize activities that nourish your mind, body, and spirit. Invest in hobbies, travel, or personal development.

- **Strengthen Existing Relationships:** Deepen connections with loved ones and cultivate new friendships. Menopause can be a time for self-discovery and building a strong support network.

- **Embrace Your Sexuality:** Menopause doesn't have to diminish your sexuality. Explore new ways of intimacy and rediscover the joy of physical connection.

- **Greater Confidence and Self-Awareness:** Years of experience have shaped you into a strong and resilient woman. Embrace your confidence and self-knowledge as you navigate this new chapter.

Menopause is an opportunity for growth, self-discovery, and empowerment. By shifting your perspective, you can embrace the positive aspects of this transition and thrive in the years ahead.

10.2 Living a Vibrant and Healthy Life After

Menopause

Here are some key strategies for living a vibrant and healthy life after menopause:

- **Maintain a Healthy Lifestyle:** A balanced diet, regular exercise, and adequate sleep are crucial for maintaining good health throughout your life.

- **Prioritize Bone Health:** Continue with your weight-bearing exercises and consider incorporating strength training routines to build and maintain bone density.

- **Schedule Regular Checkups:** Regular checkups with your doctor are essential for monitoring your health and identifying any potential concerns early. Talk to your doctor about any questions or concerns you have about menopause and its impact on your health.

- **Embrace Preventative Care:** Early detection is key. Schedule regular mammograms, colonoscopies, and other recommended screenings to maintain your well-being.

- **Stay Mentally Stimulated:** Engage in activities that challenge your mind, such as learning a new language, reading, taking a class, or volunteering.

- **Nurture Your Social Connections:** Strong social connections are crucial for emotional well-being. Stay connected with loved ones, join a club, or explore new social activities.

By prioritizing your physical and mental health, staying engaged, and maintaining strong social bonds, you can ensure a vibrant and fulfilling life after menopause.

10.3 Resources and Support Networks for Women in Menopause

You don't have to navigate menopause alone. Here are some valuable resources and support networks available to you:

- **Online Resources:** Reputable websites and online communities specifically cater to women experiencing menopause. These resources offer information, support groups, and a platform to connect with others.

- **Books and Articles:** Many informative books and articles are available on the topic of menopause.

Explore resources that address your specific needs and concerns.

- **Support Groups:** Joining a local or online menopause support group can be incredibly valuable. Connecting with other women experiencing similar changes can provide a safe space to share experiences, ask questions, and feel supported.

- **Healthcare Professionals:** Your doctor and other healthcare professionals are valuable resources for information, guidance, and potential treatment options for managing menopausal symptoms. Don't hesitate to discuss any concerns you have with your doctor.

Remember, there's no one-size-fits-all approach to menopause. Explore the resources available, find what works best for you, and build a support system that empowers you to navigate this transition with confidence.

Menopause is a natural part of a woman's life journey. By adopting a positive mindset, prioritizing your health, and accessing available resources, you can embrace this transformation and thrive in the vibrant and fulfilling years to come.

ABOUT THE AUTHOR

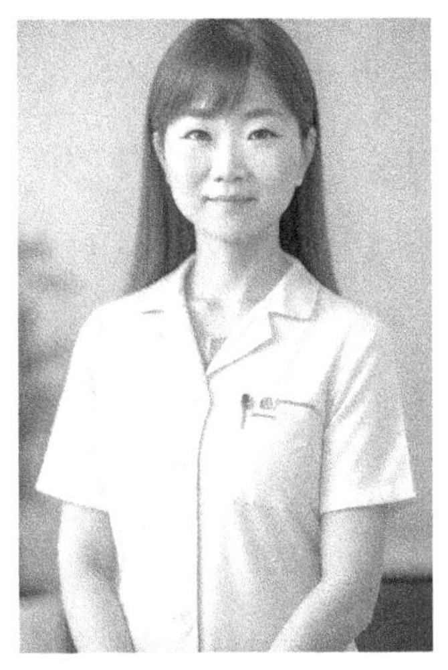

Aria Vitality is a seasoned health professional known for her holistic approach to wellness. With years of experience in nutrition, fitness, and mindfulness, she empowers individuals to achieve optimal health through personalized strategies tailored to their unique needs. Aria's passion lies in promoting overall well-being, emphasizing the importance of balanced nutrition, regular physical activity, and mental resilience. Her dedication to fostering healthy lifestyles makes her a trusted guide in the journey towards vitality and longevity.

Indeed, Aria Vitality's expertise extends to the medical realm, as she holds a doctorate in a relevant field such as naturopathic medicine or integrative health. With her medical background, she brings a comprehensive understanding of the body's physiological processes and how they intersect with lifestyle choices. Aria's multidisciplinary approach integrates traditional medical knowledge with holistic practices, allowing her to address health concerns from a holistic perspective. Whether providing personalized consultations, conducting research, or educating communities, her medical training enriches her ability to empower individuals on their journey to optimal health and well-being.